D0906377

WILLIAM F. MAAG LIBRARY
YOUNGSTOWN STATE UNIVERSITY

Y 10 5

The Ethics of Care and the Ethics of Cure: Synthesis in Chronicity

Jean Watson and Marilyn A. Ray, Editors

WITHDRAWN FROM WILLIAM F. MAAG LIBRARY YOUNGSTOWN STATE UNIVERSITY

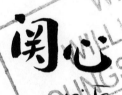

関心

CARING

関: PASSAGE
:TO THE
'心: HEART

Center for Human Caring

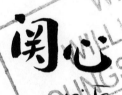

National League for Nursing • New York
Pub. No 15-2237

Copyright © 1988 by
National League for Nursing

All rights reserved. No part of this book may be
reproduced in print, or by photostatic means,
or in any other manner, without the express
written permission of the publisher.

The views expressed in this book reflect those
of the authors and do not necessarily reflect the
official views of the National League for Nursing.

ISBN 0-88737-418-2

4
8245
88

Contents

WILLIAM F. MAAG LIBRARY
YOUNGSTOWN STATE UNIVERSITY

WILLIAM F. MAAG LIBRARY
YOUNGSTOWN STATE UNIVERSITY

Contributors

Fred Abrams, MD, is associate director of the Center for Health Ethics and Policy at the University of Colorado, Denver, Colorado.

Daniel Callahan, PhD, is cofounder and director of The Hastings Center, Briarcliff Manor, New York. He is an elected member of the Institute of Medicine of the National Academy of Sciences. He is the author or editor of 25 books.

Jennifer Disabato, MS, RN, is Clinical Nurse Specialist, Pediatric/Neurosurgery Ward, The Children's Hospital, Denver, Colorado.

Sally Gadow, PhD, RN, teaches ethics at the Institute for Medical Humanities/School of Nursing, University of Texas Medical Branch, Galveston, Texas. Her areas of research and publication include the experience of illness, issues in aging, and nursing ethics.

Marilyn A. Ray, PhD, RN, is Assistant Professor, Faculty Associate, Center for Human Caring, University of Colorado School of Nursing, Denver, Colorado.

Francelyn Reeder, PhD, RSM, CNM, is Assistant Professor, Faculty Associate, Center for Human Caring, University of Colorado School of Nursing, Denver, Colorado.

Phyllis Schultz, PhD, RN, is Assistant Professor, Postdoctoral Fellow, Center for Human Caring, University of Colorado School of Nursing, Denver, Colorado.

Robert Schultz, PhD, is Associate Professor, Department of Philosophy, University of Denver.

Anna Seroka, MEd, RN, is Assistant Director of Nursing/Medicine, University Hospital, University of Colorado Health Sciences Center, Denver, Colorado.

Jean Watson, PhD, RN, FAAN, is Director, Center for Human Caring, University of Colorado Health Sciences Center School of Nursing, Denver, Colorado.

Father Paul Wicker, STB, MAS, is Consultant in Christian Ministry to Penrose Hospital and Pastor of Holy Apostles' Church, Colorado Springs, Colorado.

Preface

This work is an official publication of the University of Colorado Center for Human Caring. The Center is exploring new ways to advance the art and science of human caring. The think tank efforts in the School of Nursing range from curricular work to developing new philosophies, theories, ethics, and methods for education, research, and practices. The conference, "The Ethics of Care and the Ethics of Cure," was one of the first major conferences of the Center. It was cosponsored by The Hastings Center and the Colorado Nurses' Association. It was the first conference of its kind in helping to elucidate the issues, conflicts, and controversies associated with the traditional ethics of cure in light of the emerging dynamics and literature associated with an Ethics of Caring. In an era of aging and chronicity, how do professionals reconcile an ethic of care and cure? The Center for Human Caring Conference sought to promote an expanded ethic that accommodated a synthesis of care and cure in chronicity.

The keynote speakers, Daniel Callahan, director of the Hastings Center, and Sally Gadow of the Institute for Medical Humanities, University of Texas, Galveston, established the format with their futuristic, provocative papers followed by active practitioner-based issues, led by both national and local leaders in the field of ethics and health.

Introduction: An Ethic of Caring/Curing/ Nursing *qua* Nursing

The issues raised in this work acknowledge that the field of traditional biomedical ethics is incomplete and inadequate when it comes to issues of care and caring, especially when the elderly and chronically ill are dealt with.

Until recently, medical ethicists have ignored the field of nursing ethics, now commonly referred to as the Ethics of Caring. Indeed, an earlier view saw nursing ethics as simply a subset of medical ethics. Only in the past two to three years have traditional ethics authors begun to acknowledge that nursing ethics is a legitimate term and focus of study that refers to the ethical issues and analysis used by nurses to make ethical judgments.

Until recently, there was a trend in nursing ethics to reduce it to a common denominator. That common denominator was medicine and its traditional rationalist ethics. In other words, it has been assumed that ethical problems of nursing could be diagnosed and treated by the application of medical ethics (Gadow, 1979). However, now it can be openly acknowledged and debated that attention to medical ethics cannot substitute for comprehensive analysis of ethical human caring and curing dilemmas in nursing *qua* nursing. Such acknowledgement does not imply that medical ethics is to be discarded; it simply suggests an alternative or expanded view, or in the case of this work, a synthesis, especially in the face of chronicity.

In other words, the ideals of human caring that are rooted in receptivity, intersubjective relatedness, and human responsiveness help to counteract the medical ethic of rational principle, fairness, and equity that objictifies, detaches, and distances the professional from the subjective world of the human experience. In other words, in nursing and

1

caring we are not concerned primarily with justification through ethical principles and laws in *general*. An ethic of caring, in "contrast, ties us to the people we serve and not to the rules through which we serve them" (Noddings, 1984).

Caring is held as a moral ideal that entails a commitment to a particular end. That end is the protection and enhancement of human dignity and preservation of humanity in a chaotic, rapidly changing health care system. (Gadow, 1984; Watson, 1985).

An ethics of moral caring and curing calls out for nursing ethics that favor subjective thinking and reflection and allows time and space for seeing and feeling. In this sense, an ethic of caring has a distinct moral position; caring is attending and relating to a person in such a way that the person is protected from being reduced to the moral status of objects; likewise, nursing ethics of human care cannot be reduced to medical ethics. That is, nursing ethics should be distinguished by its philosophy and moral ideals that affirm the personal unique contextual experiences associated with human caring, inherent in nursing *qua* nursing.

In this work, both Callahan and Gadow make compelling cases for an ethics of care/caring that help to synthesize care and cure. Indeed, care is not proposed as simply a secondary fall-back position when cure is impossible. The ideas presented here help promote the discussion that we are now beyond an era where cure/curing takes precedence to an era where care/caring must take precedence. The more radical position by Gadow inverts the relationship between cure and care, designating care/caring as the highest form of commitment to patients. Caring then becomes the ethical principle or standard by which (curing) interventions are measured. Thus, with a new view presented here in these provocative papers, caring becomes the moral end, by which curing is only a means. This inversion leads to a new synthesis in care/cure issues with chronicity and elderly in our changing society. The ethics of nursing *qua* nursing, influenced by a philosophical science of caring, introduces new dimensions and challenges to traditional bioethics theory and practices.

Jean Watson, PhD, RN, FAAN
Director, Center for Human Caring
University of Colorado Health Sciences
Center School of Nursing
Denver, Colorado

REFERENCES

Callahan, D. (1987). *Setting limits: Medical goals in an aging society.* New York: Simon & Schuster.

Gadow, S. (1979). The most pressing ethical problems faced by nurses. *Advances in Nursing Science, 1*(3), 92–94.

Gadow, S. (1984). Caring as touch, technology, and truth telling. Paper presented at 1984 Research Seminar Series "Development of Nursing as a Human Science." University of Colorado School of Nursing. Denver, CO.

Noddings. N. (1984). *Caring. A feminine approach to ethics and moral education.* Berkeley, CA: University of California Press.

Watson, J. (1985). *Nursing: Human science and human care.* New York: Appleton-Century-Crofts.

CHAPTER 1
Covenant Without Cure:
Letting Go and Holding on in Chronic Illness

Sally Gadow

The ethical differences between care and cure are felt more poignantly by nurses than by any other professionals. This is made dramatically clear to me each time I receive a call from the intensive care unit for an ethics consultation on a patient around whom three groups typically are doing battle: the medical team who hope and press for cure; a family who on the patient's behalf desires release from treatment; and nurses who in the meantime—and in the middle—are committed to caring, despite the fact that theirs may be an infinite commitment without foreseeable aim or end, if the patient is able neither to die nor to recover. Without any direction in which to point their caring—either recovery or death with dignity—they are morally adrift. "Why am I doing this?" is the cry of the nurse caught in this situation.

I propose that we are responsible for being thus caught. We have set for ourselves a moral course that permits only two outcomes: either a semblance of recovery or an acceptance of death. The debate, of course, will always rage concerning the minimal level of recovery that we must accomplish in order to forestall the alternative. Since, in that view, death is the alternative, the debate is a crucial one. (Its current focus happens to be the capacity to feed oneself, with strict definitions of recovery summarized in the view "better dead than fed.")

But the tacking back and forth between death and health is not the only moral course we can set for ourselves. On that course, care is only the vessel that enables us to reach either of these ends. The alternative view that I will develop is that care is an end in itself. While it may serve

5

as a means of reaching a further state, it is always and above all a state that itself can be fully inhabited. While it may serve as a vessel for reaching a remote shore, it is at the same time and above all a vessel in which one can live even when—especially when—there is no destination in sight or in mind.

I am not proposing care as a fall-back position when cure is impossible. In much modern ethics discourse, care and cure are alternative forms of commitment to patients, so sharply distinguished that one even hears them attributed to separate professions. It is no coincidence that the two professional camps I described in the intensive care unit scenario are also different moral camps: the medical team assigned to cure, the nurses to care. So sharp can that distinction become that we find situations in which they seem mutually exclusive: The classic case is that in which cure requires painful treatment, while the deliberate causing of pain is—for most patients and nurses—difficult to reconcile with care. In most such cases (either because patients desire cure or because the curemongers in the situation happen also to be the decision makers), cure is elected, and care is set aside. In the opposite situation, such as chronic illness, the either/or operates the other way: When cure is impossible, professionals judge that nothing but care can be their role.

It is precisely not this "nothing but" meaning of care that I am proposing. With that meaning, the most dedicated nurses understandably find themselves unbearably frustrated with chronic care, because the "nothing but" view clearly is premised upon *cure* as the most worthwhile aim of health care (health cure?).

In my discussion I will invert that relationship between cure and care, designating care as the highest form of commitment to patients, encompassing as many different expressions of concern for patient well-being as we are imaginative enough to devise; the frustrating situations will be those in which the scope of our concern is limited to a single treatable problem, in the care for which there is nothing to do but provide the remedy. There is, in other words, *nothing but cure* that we can offer, if the situation is so constricted that the infinitely more encompassing breadth of care either cannot be offered or received.

A NEW RELATIONSHIP BETWEEN CARE AND CURE

Exactly what is the care that I am elevating above even cure as the supreme covenant into which nurse and patient can enter? Let me try to define it, then illustrate it.

The covenant of care I have in mind is the commitment to alleviating another's vulnerability. If that seems so simple and general as to include everything a health professional does, let me hasten to point out that the treatment measures that first come to mind as the most dramatic efforts to alleviate vulnerability—for example, surgical interventions—are actually the least consistent with the concept I am proposing. That is because they achieve their effect through the exercise of power by one person over another, and the exercise of power always *increases* the vulnerability of the one over whom it is exercised, no matter what benevolent purpose the power serves. Let me suggest that all measures directed toward cure of a condition (as distinct from prevention or accommodation) require the exercise of power and thus are the most difficult to include within the realm of care. They must be included, in order for them to be morally valid and not examples of torture. And they can be included, provided that the powerlessness created by the treatment is regarded as a vulnerability (in this case iatrogenic) that calls as urgently for alleviation as the initial disease-induced vulnerability.

My position, in short, by defining care as the alleviation of vulnerability, has the perhaps surprising effect of regarding cure as morally problematic at best and immoral at worst. Only in the context of care can the overpowering of one person by another that cure entails be redeemed. This inverts our usual framework, in which we regard acute, treatable illness as the morally clearest situation with the fewest issues and chronic illness as the morally blurred situation in which the variety of interventions possible, the eventual futility of any of them, compounded at times by the veiled character of the condition and the patient's wavering motivation, make the morally right response almost impossible to discern. In the view I am proposing, the opposite is the case. Acute, straightforwardly reversible conditions create the greater moral problem, exactly because of the unequivocal effectiveness of the external intervention and thus the degree of power exerted over the individual to achieve that effect. Chronic illness, on the other hand, offers few possibilities to wield that degree of power over a patient's condition and thus less temptation to risk violating the covenant of care by creating new vulnerability in the person with whom we have covenanted to alleviate vulnerability.

In this framework, *care* is the ethical principle or standard by which interventions are measured. Interventions as extreme as cure that succeed through power alone are the most difficult to justify by the moral standard of care. In the usual view, of course, *cure* is the standard, the overriding goal, and care is nothing but a means toward that end. In my view, care is the moral end, and cure is only a means to that end; more often it is a detour from which we may not find our way back to the patient.

WILLIAM F. MAAG LIBRARY
YOUNGSTOWN STATE UNIVERSITY

DONALD: A DIFFICULT SYNTHESIS OF CARE AND CURE

To illustrate the position I am proposing, let me describe a case in which I find the synthesis of care and cure the most difficult because of the alienation that cure seemingly entailed and the agonizing vulnerability that treatment created in a man already overwhelmed to the last degree by his situation. My point in analyzing this case is not to argue that cure measures are in themselves immoral because they overpower and thus violate patients. I want only to suggest that they become immoral when the power through which cure is achieved creates a degree of vulnerability so extreme that no human caring can assuage it.

The case is that of Donald Cowart, about whom many of you have already read. Ten years ago Donald was seriously burned, then treated with interventions covering the spectrum of burn care from tubbing and grafting to reconstructive surgery. Throughout his months and eventually years of "cure" or "care" (let us not yet decide how to categorize his treatment), he refused to give his consent, and for that reason his case has become a classic in the medical ethics literature. Two videotapes of him have been made and thousands of words written discussing the issue of treatment without consent. That issue, however, I am going to disregard on the grounds that the issue concerning us today—the synthesis of care and cure—is just as profoundly difficult when consent *is* given. Consent affects only one moral dimension of a case. Another equally important dimension is that addressed by the concept of care I have proposed, that is, the covenant to alleviate vulnerability. Consent has no effect upon the obligation not to intensify or create new vulnerability: Patients do not consent to indignity; they consent to specific procedures. Even if Donald had consented to every intervention, the obligation to care would not have been cancelled, and his plight would still illustrate the extraordinarily difficult synthesis of cure and care.

Donald's situation—as we meet him 10 years ago—is that of a person burned, blinded, without use of his hands, and regularly subjected to excruciating interventions. His vulnerability may be more extreme than that of other patients, but his situation is especially instructive for that reason. It illuminates the basic moral problem present in all cases in which we seek to reconcile cure and care: the problem of crossing the chasm between the patient's intensified embodiment and the professional's disembodiment. That chasm we must examine carefully, because the possibility of crossing it is the only means of alleviating vulnerability, and measures that make it uncrossable thereby make care impossible and cure unethical.

The chasm is the existential distance between patient and nurse: the

difference between having the body as one's only—and entirely nega-
tive—sphere of existence versus freely functioning without regard for
the possible torments of embodiment. Experience normally moves easily
between these two realms, an individual alternately becoming so absorbed
by activities that the body is forgotten, then being recalled to it by hunger,
for example, or fatigue. In Donald's situation the two realms of physical
existence that usually interweave within one person are divided. His own
overwhelming reality is embodiment, while those who care for him are,
in relation to him, disembodied. How this gulf arises will differ in each
case; Donald's case summarizes virtually all of the ways in which it can
happen.

First, the avenues that normally lead a person out of the body and
away from its intensity—the eyes and the hands—are for him perma-
nently closed. The eyes and hands are our most developed means of
both receiving and altering the world. Vision can passively register as
well as actively edit the objects around us; between people the eyes are
even more powerful, able to intrude as well as deflect intrusion. The
hands are the material version of this almost metaphysical power. The
original tool and still the supreme one for many tasks, the hand sym-
bolizes the human power of reconstructing the world. Together, eyes
and hands represent freedom from the body's tyranny. Without them
the world is an indifferent other, the body a prison.

For Donald and many burned patients that helplessness is emphasized
by prolonged nakedness. The result is the paradoxical openness that
nakedness enforces, combined with the isolation of a closed interiority
without eyes or hands. Singly, these conditions might not be overwhelming. Naked but sighted, Donald could fend off others' gaze with his eyes.
Or blind, he could hide from other eyes, were he capable of covering
his nakedness. But naked, blind, and helpless, he is wholly submerged
in the body. For others too, therefore, his body is his entire being, fully
exposed to them, unprotected and public, unable to flee or to shield itself.

For himself as well as those caring for him, Donald's existence is defined
by the body. But, unlike him, they are disembodied. In her study of
pain, Elaine Scarry notes, "The one with authority and power has no
body for his inferiors" (Scarry, 1985). In clinical situations the discrep-
ancy between the hidden body of the professional and the exposed,
emphasized body of the patient is not just an expression of power: It is
one of its sources. In Donald's blindness that power is magnified, since
his nurses cannot be seen by him at all. Nor can he touch them, clasp
their hands in his. They touch him at their discretion, often gloved or
with instruments, reminding him of his own body's presence rather than

theirs. In every respect, his embodiment is intensified to the highest degree, while theirs is omitted entirely from their relationship to him. They are voices with tools but not bodies.

The power that instruments and tools represent, the power of overcoming both the body's given limits and the given forms of the world, further widens the chasm. Without hands or tools, Donald has no means of physically affecting his world. But because of that very inability, he provides to others almost unlimited possibility in that regard through their reconstruction of his body. That which is forbidden to him is their freedom, the escape from embodiment through making, remaking, and affecting the world. The destruction of that possibility in him has directly increased it for them. His loss is their gain because he is their gain: It is his body through which they transcend their own. The remaking of the human body—in even the most minor ways—can be considered the supreme artifice, the highest art, but although he provides the material for that ultimate recreating, it is a project in which he cannot participate. It would be better if he were not even present consciously. His agony is a distraction for those who must with such painstaking and paingiving attentiveness accomplish that artifice.

With the causing of pain, the gulf between patient and caregiver widens almost beyond crossing: "Whatever their spatial proximity, there are no two experiences farther apart than suffering and inflicting pain" (Scarry, 1985). The inflicting of pain for any purpose requires disassociation from one's own body in order not to suffer with the person in pain. In circumstances where much suffering is witnessed and much inflicted, as in long and agonizing treatment, protecting the caregiver from pain is a necessity. That protection is afforded only by disassociation from one's own body in order not to emphatically recognize the patient's pain. So crucial, in fact, is that disassociation that it accounts for the paradox in which it is sometimes easier to increase someone's pain (as in child battering) than simply to witness it and suffer helplessly in response. Causing pain in another becomes a means of preventing it in oneself, because in deliberately inflicting it on another, a decisive repudiation of one's own body is accomplished.

Through Donald's other conditions—the absence of eyes, hands, clothes, even skin—he becomes desperately vulnerable, even before any pain is inflicted, and the distance between his overwhelming embodiment and the professional's disembodiment is vast indeed. But with the inflicting of pain, the gulf widens to become almost infinite. This sudden widening is not due just to the violation that pain always is felt to be, producing in us a vulnerability as excruciating as the pain itself. In addition, and regardless of whether the pain has been consented to or not, the distance between patient and nurse becomes through pain an abyss, because the nurse, in order to accomplish that violation, must repudiate her own vulnerability, that is, her own embodiment. Up to this point the chasm between them was a function of Donald's condition. At this point, it becomes a function of the nurse's condition, the now explicitly erected wall between the nurse and her own body.

The last possibility for alleviating patients' vulnerability is destroyed when nurses become invulnerable—thus the danger that causing pain marks a point of no return in the departure from the moral standard of care I have proposed. It matters not whether the pain is for therapeutic purposes (we assume it is) or whether patients have consented (we hope they have). What matters is that an almost unbridgeable abyss has opened between patient and nurse, between their utterly opposite stages of embodiment. Unless ways can be found to alter both of those states, each in the direction of the other, the alleviation of vulnerability is impossible because the gulf is uncrossable. This means, in short, that care is impossible, and efforts to cure—outside the context of care—are unethical.

BRIDGING THE GULF

For care to become possible in Donald's situation, two changes are needed. He must be assisted to reach beyond the imprisoning body, while those caring for him must find ways of reinhabiting their own bodies in relation to his.

Donald has no physical means of extending himself beyond the body, but he has speech. The voice is his form of transcendence, his projection of self beyond body and suffering. But the transcending of embodiment through speech would be impossible even if—like many patients—he were without words, provided that someone spoke "with his voice," expressing for him the moral claim that vulnerability makes upon us. That advocacy is possible only when the advocate's voice arises, like vulnerability itself, from the depths of embodiment. He cannot be represented by the language of bodiless advocates. This leads to the second change required for care to be possible, the need for his caregivers to transcend their disembodiment, to experience the world from within the body as he does. How is that bridge to be built across the gulf between them, even when—especially when—pain is inflicted?

The bridge that will make care possible consists of their uncovering to themselves and, thus, to Donald their own embodiment. Since it is not the mere fact but the meanings of having a body that their disembodiment denies, literal disclosure of the body misses the point. Clinical practices that mimic self-disclosure—professionals shedding official garb, sitting on a patient's bed, letting patients examine them—fail for that reason. Instead of divulging personal meanings of embodiment, they are an exercise in disembodiment, a display of the extent to which the body can be bared without the person "inside" being found out. The practices are not without risk since they flirt with embodiment, but they are a gratuitous flirting, freely initiated, freely ended, a charade performed in the face of the patient's genuine, unfree embodiment.

While Donald's blindness makes literal for him the disembodied state of his nurses, recovery of sight would not alter that state in his perception, just as the charade of professional familiarity toward patients proves to them no more than they know already, that is, the abstract fact that professionals have bodies. The proof of embodiment comes not through seeing or touching a body to confirm its existence as an *object*. Rather, the evidence must be of a different type, evidence that the professional's body has the same compelling *subjective* reality as the patient's body.

How is that subjective reality to be conveyed? How is Donald to discover that his caregivers too are embodied and vulnerable?

One means is through their revealing to him the vulnerability that summarizes for them, as for him, the body's significance, disclosing to him their own anguish, fear, and bewilderment. It is the attempt at disembodiment that has made these seem like purely psychological states, unrelated to physical experience, when in fact their origin lies in limitations inherent in the body. A bodiless being is invulnerable; thus, vulnerability confided by one person to another is a testimony to the body's subjectivity.

The second testimony, enlarging infinitely upon the first, is the transmuting of vulnerability into its opposite, its alleviation. Thus, from the nurse's own vulnerability emerge an intensity of empathic regard and a corresponding refinement of physical ministration in which the smallest gesture or the least touch is capable of easing the patient's suffering. In that form of care is found the positive pole in the dialectic of embodiment, the fact that vulnerability in the nurse is *enabling*, and thus that in the patient vulnerability is itself vulnerable to care: Even at its worst, it can be assuaged, but only through the forms of care that an empathic—because it is embodied—imagination creates.

Bridging the chasm in these ways removes none of the moral ambiguity of inflicting pain. But it relieves the urgency for erecting moral frameworks in which to justify pain. In a situation such as I have defined cure to be, consisting of one person unilaterally acting upon another, justification is of course essential—although even absolute justification, were such available, would do nothing toward alleviating the vulnerability created by the pain. On the contrary, when justification is predicated on the agent's moral certainty (one form of invulnerability), the possibility is lost for alleviating vulnerability in the patient.

As long as Donald and his nurses remain mutually engaged in each other's vulnerability and its alleviation, the existential distance between them diminishes. The fact that they inflict pain and he experiences it describes one dimension of their reality. But beyond that, he is assisted to project himself outside the torment of embodiment, and they in turn are able to emerge from behind their disembodiment. Their bodies as well as their voices answer his voice and body. The moment that mutuality is abandoned and the chasm reopened, then power again is unilateral, and cure is unethical.

LYMAN: CARING AS RITUAL

The case of Donald Cowart illustrates the nature of the difficulty in achieving a synthesis of cure and care. The case of Lyman, in contrast, illustrates that synthesis is achieved in the supremely modest, even mundane, care a patient receives from his nurse. Listen to Lyman's own words describing the small ceremony in which the vulnerability of both patient and nurse is acknowledged and its alleviation celebrated.

> Already we have a comfortable rut, we go through habitual motions whose every stage is reassuring. While she starts the bath water, I wheel my chair into the bedroom, just beside the bathroom door. We don't bother with the crutches. She helps her grotesque doll to stand up, and it clings to her while her gnarled hands, the end joints twisted almost at right angles, fumble with zippers and buttons. . . . The water is so hot that it makes the stump prickle and smart, but it must be that hot if it is to ease the aches away enough to permit sleep. Painfully she wallows down on her knees and without diffidence soaps and rinses me all over. Her crooked fingers drag across the skin stiff as twigs. Her doll sits stiffly, pointed straight ahead at the fixtures that emerge from the wall. When she is finished she bends far over and guides its arms around her neck. Then she rears upward, and up it comes, naked and pink, her hairy baby, its stump bright red.
>
> Holding it, clucking and murmuring as she works, she towels it down as far as the knees, and then she takes it around the waist and tilts it upon her great bosom and rotates until its leg, bent to miss the tub's rim, can straighten down on the mat. Pressing it against her as intimate as husband, she towels the rest of it and eases it into the chair and wheels it to the bed. . . . Now the pajamas, delicious to the chilling skin, and the ease backward until the body that has been upright too long is received by mattress and pillows. She sets the telephone close, she tucks up the covers. Finally she waddles over to the cabinet by the desk and gets the bottle and two glasses, and we have a comfortable nightcap together. (Stegner, 1971)

LETTING GO AND HOLDING ON

It will have become clear by now that holding on and letting go are concepts that make sense only within an ethic devoted to cure. In that model we face often agonizing ethical choices predicated upon the difference between continuing to struggle for recovery and giving in to death.

In the ethical model I have described, based upon the covenant of care, the crucial distinction is not that between health and death, but that of alleviating versus intensifying vulnerability. The central moral choice that emerges here is not whether to hold onto or let go of life, but whether to hold onto or let go of the special covenantal relationship of caring. Giving up on cure and giving in to death need not mean letting go of that relationship. On the contrary, single-minded, morally certain commitment to cure may compromise if not sacrifice the relationship more surely than a decision to let go of every hope for cure. We know this empathically if only through contrasting the often crippling assault that life-prolonging treatment can represent and, on the other hand, the exquisitely sensitive tenderness with which the dying person often is cared for.

The greatest ethical task of the nurse is reconciling those two extremes, maintaining a relationship in which the chasm is never uncrossable, where no assault is permitted unless it can be redeemed, not by its future effect but by the immediate, present caring of the nurse who, because she has not let go of her own vulnerability, is able to reach across and hold on to patients in their vulnerability. That holding on represents a rich synthesis—of cure and care, of nurse and patient, of embodiment and transcendence. Without question, such a synthesis is the highest moral accomplishment and the most arduous task we face in nursing.

REFERENCES

Scarry, E. (1985). *The body in pain: The making and unmaking of the world.* New York: Oxford University Press, p. 210.

Scarry, E. (1985). *The body in pain: The making and unmaking of the world.* New York: Oxford University Press, p. 47.

Stegner, W. (1971). *The angle of repose.* New York: Doubleday, pp. 103–104.

CHAPTER 2
Setting Limits:
Medical Goals in an Aging Society

Daniel Callahan

The title of this session is identical with that of a new book I will be publishing. Let me give you some background on that book. Ever since I have been working in the field of biomedical ethics, I have been particularly interested in the question of technology and how we understand it, how we control it, and how we get it to serve human ends. The first instance of this was an early interest in prenatal diagnosis, artificial reproduction, and then eventually organ transplantation and a wide range of other issues.

Beginning a few years ago, I became interested in the question of the allocation of resources in general. It is obvious that we are beginning to have severe financial and other problems with the health care system. I was particularly interested in the role that technology has played in the escalation of cost and began asking the question: Where is this whole system going? Is the system full of contradictions? On the one hand, we would like to find ways to control costs, and various efforts are under way to do that. But, on the other hand, there is a great eagerness to continue developing new technologies that inevitably drive up the cost.

As I was thinking about that issue, I became more interested in the question of the care of the aged. That was brought about by certain things that caught my attention and also impinged upon our attention at The Hastings Center. First, about four years ago, I became interested in data that were beginning to come out in the medical literature that raised rather disturbing questions about the allocation of resources. This data showed that almost 30 percent of Medicare funds go to 5 percent of the elderly—those who are in the last year of life. In other words, a great amount of money is spent on the dying, and the question was raised of whether it is a wise expenditure or not. We looked very carefully into that problem, and it turned out, fortunately, that there was less there than appeared on the surface. Because, as you know, it is very difficult to determine who is in fact dying, the issue did not turn out to be quite as significant as was our first impression.

However, shortly after that, another debate broke out, one that sometimes carries the label of the intergenerational equity problem. This debate came about in great part because of a presidential address given by the demographer Samuel Preston in 1984 before the Population Association of America. He presented some very disturbing statistics. The gist of his statistics was that, over the past decade or so, there has been a very sharp shift of public resources from the young to the old. He showed that those over the age of 65 get from six to seven times as much federal money as those under the age of 18.

Moreover, when one looks at the history of Social Security or Medicare, it is possible to see that when Medicare was introduced in 1965, some 35 percent of the elderly were under the poverty line—and an even larger proportion in 1935, when Social Security was introduced. By the mid-1980s, however, that figure was down to 12 or 14 percent. The economic status of the elderly had appreciably increased over the years. Meanwhile, the status of the young has deteriorated; in the mid-1960s some 15 percent of families with children lived under the poverty line, but by the mid-1980s that figure had risen to over 21 percent.

A third issue was also noted, one that was less prominent and less controversial, but nonetheless significant. With the exception of the birth control pill and neonatal intensive care units, most high-technology medicine benefits an older rather than a younger population. Moreover, a great many technologies originally introduced to help the younger generations have seen a kind of age creep, so that the average user's age is going up. Dialysis was originally introduced to help those between the ages of 15 and 45. Now some 30 percent of those on dialysis are over the age of 65.

These three different incidents were, when taken together, rather striking. They suggested to me that there is the beginning of some fundamental questioning about how we allocate resources to the elderly and also about how we think about the future of the old in relationship to the future of the young. This stimulated me to begin thinking about health care for the elderly as case studies in allocation and high-technology medicine. The more I thought about the matter, the more it seemed obvious to me that—given the many things I have mentioned so far, and given the pressures for greater economy and efficiency in the health care delivery system—we are going to have to ask a basic question about what is a fair amount of health care to give to the elderly.

What is a reasonable proportion of our health care resources to provide to the elderly? As you can see, it is certainly a problem of allocation. But it is something more as well. It is also a question about the future of the health care system and about the goals of medicine. There are projections that show that by the year 2030 or so, we could be spending half of all health care money in this country on the elderly. However, that would make no sense, given the health care needs of other age groups, not to mention other social needs as well. It would be a simply staggering figure.

We have to begin again and ask some basic questions about the health care system, about the meaning and purpose of medicine, and about the significance of aging itself. What are proper goals? Given the fact that medicine can spend an enormous and constantly increasing amount of money on the elderly, care of the elderly is thus the endless frontier of medicine. It is, in fact, an infinite frontier. We can spend forever if we deal with all the conditions of the elderly, and there will always be new conditions to deal with. Is it proper for medicine simply to go on with no sense of limits, and no limits or an ultimate direction?

What are the proper goals of aging? To talk about the goals of aging may seem like a difficult question, but what I mean is this: Now that medicine can keep people alive longer and both extend life and improve the quality of life, how should we conceive of the future of old age? This is an interesting question because there are some groups, particularly some of the aging advocacy groups, that want to see old age as a whole new stage of life. They would have us make of old age the beginning of a new life.

But the question is whether that is an appropriate goal. Is it appropriate in the face of some significant unbalancing of allocations between the old and the young? If we think that old age ought to be the beginning of a new life, that we ought to conquer this endless frontier, then we can spend an enormous amount of money, with no end in sight, and also in the process do a fair degree of harm to other social needs.

Such considerations led me to conclude that we have to set limits somewhere, that medicine would have to control its ambitions on this new frontier. It cannot simply and infinitely try for more and more. At the same time, I concluded that it didn't make sense to think of aging, or old age, as the beginning of a new life at all—that, in fact, there is more to the traditional wisdom that the purpose of old age is to live out a reasonably satisfactory life, but also to prepare for one's death. But old age ought also to become a period when the old—so far as they can—begin to think of what they are going to leave to the next generation. Hence, I argue that the primary obligation of the old is not to themselves, but to the young and to the generations to come. Part of the stewardship of being old is that one must worry about what comes after, and that one is responsible in some significant sense for the fate of the next generation.

But how are we to set limits, if we agree that we should not go on indefinitely in the present direction, and that we risk harm to others by even trying to do so? I came up with a proposal that will not please many people, but I believe it makes sense. It may, in fact, provide us with our only realistic option. The elderly ought not, beyond a certain age, be entitled to government reimbursement for life-extending medical care, particularly high technology medical care. We should always relieve pain and suffering, but I do not believe we are morally obligated to provide everything that medical technology offers by way of life extension.

We have a ridiculous situation in this country where one cannot get decent long-term care at affordable prices, or without the risk of making oneself a pauper. One can get money for the acute care necessary to save one's life from a heart attack, but not for the long-term or home care that might be necessary for the months or years following that attack. That is a very serious imbalance.

What is a decent lifespan, and how much of it do we actually need to live a decent life? Indeed, this is a difficult question to answer. However, in my attempt to formulate an answer, I started with simple, familiar experiences everyone is aware of.

First, we have the experience that most people who are old or are at least approaching old age do not say they are looking for immortality, at least immortality on earth, or an infinite life for their body. Instead, they say they want to be independent, that they do not want to be a burden to their family, that they want to die humanely, and that they do not want to die surrounded by tubes and machines, or in the back room of a nursing home.

Second, at funerals of those over 80, there is very little weeping, unless the deceased endured an unusually painful death. If someone has lived out a reasonably decent and long life, has raised a family, and has done most of the things that people get a chance to do in a human life, we ordinarily take death at that point to be a natural event. As it turns out, most of the world's religious traditions express a similar perception, which explains something of our reaction to the death of those who are 80 or older.

As I tried to collect these thoughts, I attempted to determine what might count as a natural lifespan—an acceptable and tolerable length of life. Such a determination, it seemed to me, might provide some foundation for public policy.

How much life do you need to live a good life? In one sense, no matter at what age we die, it is going to be too early. There will always be things undone. If you live to be 150, but have loving relationships with other people, it is still going to be too short a life. You will have to break off those relationships. There will always be more books to read, more places to see, more people to meet, more experiences to be had. But that is the case regardless of how long one lives. On the other hand, many people who have unhappy lives are not going to be made happier by getting 10 more years of life.

It was that way of thinking that prompted the idea of using age as a basis of limiting health care. I believe it can be a meaningful standard, that it can be a fair standard, and that it can be a standard that will much better than at present ensure an adequate distribution of resources between and among age groups. Even if we had infinite resources, I am not certain that an effort to continually extend the average human life span would be a good thing. Old age will be made meaningful by the social and individual meaning we bring to it, not simply by better medical technology. We must set limits. A decent life and a good old age seem to me adequate goals to aim for and goals that are feasible. As a good and sensible balance, we can provide a much higher quality of care for the elderly, but this must be done at the price of limiting life-extending technology.

CHAPTER 3

Discussion Group Summary: Hospitals Under Stress— The Compromising of Care

Fred Abrams

Perhaps we ought to be thinking strictly about medical care when we talk about hospitals under stress. Nevertheless, the discussion soon devolves to the raw issues of money and law. These issues are not totally separate, either.

The first economic pressures, of course, result in the problem of patient transfers—which is a euphemism for patient dumping. The articles that deal with this topic show increases in the number of patients transferred each year since various cost-cutting methods by the federal government and private insurance companies were started around 1983.

What were the demographics of this dumping? Eighty to ninety percent of the patients in all of these studies were black or Hispanic, and largely unemployed. Three percent of the transfers had private insurance— meaning 97 percent were uninsured, or were covered by Medicare or Medicaid. There was an even more subtle reason to transfer, and that was for a diagnosis that was not profitable.

The Joint Commission on Accreditation of Hospitals has some regulations on this matter. It says that access to hospitals must be impartial, regardless of race, creed, ethnic group, national origin, or ability to pay. The American College of Emergency Physicians says that emergency care must be given without regard to ability to pay. And the ethics code of the American Medical Association states, "No one can be rejected at a hospital where they appear for emergency treatment, unless that hos-

---

This paper is an edited version of an informal talk by Dr. Abrams designed to summarize topics of concern under discussion.

pital cannot give the treatment." Nothing is said about stabilizing patients or whether they can afford treatment or not. It isn't "send them on down to the city hospital if everything's okay," but instead, "if you can take care of them, you're obliged to take care of them if they appear at your hospital."

Of course there are two sides to this question, too, because some hospitals in certain areas of a city would probably be overburdened with this kind of problem. Therefore, it's not all "the nasty old hospital is turning people away"; it is more like "what are we going to do about this in an equitable manner?"

Twenty-two states now have laws that stipulate that emergency care must be given, at least until a patient is stabilized. There was a case in Texas about two years ago, in which a young boy had a fracture, was "stabilized," sent down to the city hospital, had his open reduction there, had some increased limitation of motion and action—then sued the initial hospital and won in the state of Texas with a very strongly worded decision that said, in essence, "When you've got an emergency, you've got to take care of it."

What has the federal government done about this? In 1986, it actually passed a federal law against dumping. Any hospital that accepts Medicare may not dump an emergency patient or a woman in active labor. What's wrong with the law? It doesn't define "emergency" or "stabilization," and there is no established means to monitor or enforce the law. It is on the books, but unless someone has taken the initiative to pursue this law, so far its effect is unknown.

In the meantime, $600 million was cut from Medicaid from 1981 to 1983, when most of these studies were done. And, interestingly enough, in 1984 profits in private hospitals were higher than at any time in the previous 20 years. I think that many private hospitals were getting ready to lose money, but they didn't do it that year and ended up practicing for the upcoming year. However, it is important that there are incentives for dumping, and they are cuts in government money to cover the indigent. It's difficult to fault the private hospitals, which have to stay alive. And while the community may press its legislature to pass laws that prohibit dumping, I did not see many legislatures passing those laws and, at the same time, saying, "However, we are going to add a sales tax to reimburse those hospitals for taking care of the indigent patient." There was not a good balance.

Hospital joint ventures with doctors, nurses, physiotherapists, social workers, psychologists, and psychiatrists are the source of another economic dilemma, and while there can be several kinds of problems, they basically revolve around the ethical issue of conflict of interest. And, again, the law has stepped into this. Some states say that physicians involved in a joint venture may not refer patients to it at all; other states say that if they do, they must make a full disclosure of their affiliation. Obviously, the concern is that referrals will be channeled some place where it's profitable for the referrer, which may not necessarily be the best solution for the patient.

Some of the ethical problems we're running into really are a result of our social schizophrenia: We are both egalitarians and capitalists, and that's where the trouble lies. If a wealthy person purchases some new technology, pretty soon the poorer people want it, and our philosophy up to very recently has been that you can't say no, because we believe in egalitarian principles. Our alternative is that you could either deny it to everybody or give it to everybody, and so far we think it should be given to everybody because we feel you can't prevent someone who can afford it from buying whatever medical care they want. Interestingly enough, there have been some strange things that happened in California in the same year that a quarter million people were cut off the Medicaid roles. Liver transplants became an insurance benefit, which meant insurance companies had to pay for livers for a few people while another quarter million went without medical care. These are the kinds of pressures and rationing that we face in this country from a hit-or-miss type of method, depending on who gets the legislator's ear at any particular time.

I spoke about economics, and I would like to speak briefly about the impact of law. Although I reiterate that they are both overlapping, I'd like to speak about the pressures on the hospital from the law.

The first pressure that we saw very clearly was back in the initial Baby Doe case in Bloomington, Indiana, where a Down's syndrome child with a tracheo-esophogeal fistula was not operated on to repair the fistula. Clearly, the child could not be fed by a tube because food would go into the lungs, and, clearly, the only chance the child had to survive was surgical procedure. The issue of consent was explained to the parents in such a way that they and the court were advised that the Down's syndrome child would have no quality in life whatsoever, that he would be a vegetable, and that he would never relate to his parents—a very grim picture, indeed. However, two successive courts relied upon the opinion to uphold the parents' right to refuse surgery, and while an appeal was being formulated, the child died. That raised a great hue and cry across the country, because it was falsely concluded that if this was happening in Bloomington, it probably happened a thousand times a day in Chicago, Denver, and New York. Investigations proved that it didn't happen a thousand times a day—not even once a day, and probably not even once a year. Hordes of investigators came streaming down on various hospitals, investigated scores of cases, disrupted innumerable nurseries across the country, and found not a single case that violated regulations which were interpreted to say you may not discriminate against someone because he or she is handicapped. Ultimately, the courts decided that that "handicap law" was not intended by Congress to regulate medical care anyway, and it was thrown out.

While this and a second case in Stonybrook, New York, were unfolding, various interested groups came up with suggested guidelines, which say that any child born with a serious handicap must be treated, with three exceptions: if the child is irreversibly comatose; if the child has a number of conditions, and treating one of them will not keep the child from dying anyway; and if treatment would be virtually futile and, thus, would be inhumane to pursue. Regardless of the above three conditions, all children must have appropriate nutrition and hydration, and, therefore, one cannot allow a Down's syndrome child to starve to death in the nursery, as happened in Bloomington.

In summary, we have two great pressures that lead to the compromise of care: economic and legal. We are the buffers between the community and the patients, and doctors and nurses ought to feel they are the patients' advocates and not the community's representatives. With those caveats, I think we all have our work cut out for us in making sure that both economic pressures and legal pressures do not compromise good care in hospitals.

CHAPTER 4
Discussion Group Summary: Setting the Limits: Medical Goals in an Aging Society

Daniel Callahan

What is it that medicine ought to be aiming for in the care of the elderly? Given that question, I wondered how we are going to think about the meaning and purpose of aging itself. So I came up with a double question—where ought medicine go in care of the elderly? And what should it aspire to, what should its goals be?

Given the fact that medicine can spend an enormous and constantly increasing amount of money on the elderly, in one sense care of the elderly is the endless frontier of medicine. We have become fairly expert at taking care of the younger generations, and we have gotten mortality and morbidity down. And there are always new ways to go; you can think of patient groups that need more. But with the elderly, it is infinite. We can spend forever if we deal with all the conditions of the elderly now through some medical miracle. Also, we can be sure that there are going to be other conditions to take their place. That is the endless frontier.

Therefore, the question is: Ought medicine simply have as its goal just going on and on and doing everything possible so that no boundaries and no limits are set? Should it do so regardless of the cost? Some would say it should. They would say we should respect the elderly, and medicine should always try to save life and relieve suffering, therefore, go for it. That's one point of view, particularly among many aging advocates. They decry the very notion of setting limits or instituting controls. They think it's a subtle way of discriminating against the elderly, so they don't even like this kind of talk.

A related question, however, is what do we want to think of as the proper goals of aging? Now that medicine can keep people alive longer and to some extent improve the quality of life, how should we conceive of the future of old age? This is an interesting question because there are some groups—particularly some of the aging advocacy groups—that want to see old age as really a whole new stage of life that is now opening up for the first time with the help of medicine to be something it never was before. There's a wonderful radio ad for the magazine *Modern Maturity*, published by the American Association of Retired Persons, which talks about old age as the beginning of a new life. That is an interesting idea. It used to be that it was the end of the old life; now it is the beginning of a new one. However, you can only say that you understand this if you think of investing large sums of money to maintain health in old age.

All of this led me to conclude, first, that we had to set limits somewhere—that this was not a viable way to go—and, second, that medicine would have to control its ambitions on this new frontier in some way. It couldn't just infinitely try to do more and more. At the same time, I began to think it didn't make sense to think of aging, or old age, as the beginning of a new life at all—that, in fact, there is more to the kind of traditional wisdom that says the purpose of old age is, on the one hand, to live out a reasonably satisfactory life, and, on the other, to prepare for one's death. One is at the end of life and at a period when it is time to begin to think of what one is going to bequeath to the next generation. Hence, I argue that the primary obligation of the old is not to themselves, but instead to the young and the days to come, and that part of the stewardship of being old and the inheritors of this society is that one must then think of what's coming after one and what one ought leave to that next generation.

All of this became more concrete as I tried to think through the policy. If I started with the viewpoint that we have to set limits to the notion of what old age ought to be and limits to medicine's aspirations on this frontier, then I asked: How will that work out in terms of policy? And I came up with a proposal that will not please many people, but I think it still makes sense: We may have to decide that beyond a certain point the elderly cannot receive life-extending medical care. The way we set the limit is: We simply say that you will reach a point in your life where you will always be eligible to have your suffering relieved and pain dealt with, but you will no longer be eligible, at least under Medicare, to have the kind of creeping immortality prevalent today.

Currently, we have an enormous bias that if someone has a coronary—and that can get very expensive even if you're 99—you can get care in an intensive care unit, regardless of your prospects for extended life after that. At the same time, though, we have a ridiculous situation where you cannot get good long-term care. Therefore, it might be better to have a heart attack if you want to get money from taxpayers; if you need long-term care or home care, then you're in real trouble. That seems strange. In trying to work all of this through, I sought to ask two questions: What is it that we really need in life as we try to think about the health care system and as we try to think about old age approaching? Beyond that, especially, what do we owe each other, in terms of providing health care and support? In response, I began to consider the idea of what I called a natural life span. By natural life span, I mean how much life do we need to live an adequately decent life? How many years?

As I tried to think this through—what my count is of what I called a natural life span: an acceptable, tolerable length of life—it seemed that that might provide some foundation for public policy. If we could say that is one way of limiting expenditures on an infinity of aspirations, we certainly could say that our task as a society and our obligation toward each other is to see that we all avoid premature death and live out a natural life span. We may debate how long that is, but I would say it reaches into the late 70s or early 80s. There are always cases of the man who started running marathons at 85; my mother was a painter who started painting at 75. There are always people who start things late in life, but I don't believe we owe each other, through the Medicare system, continuation of life in general through expensive high technology and medicine simply because there are some people who take up things late in life.

Therefore, if one asks, "How much life do you really need?" the answer is necessarily, "more life." But it's not clear to me that more life is the essence of a happy life. In fact, the relationship between a happy life and a long life is not clear at all.

If you try to think of social policy in this way, then we might ask, do our social or mutual obligations to each other stop once we have helped each other to reach a natural life span? If so, then we have a basis for limiting health care, which is a basis that does not depend upon medical technology. The standard answer in medicine to the question of allocation of health care is that you should only do it on the basis of need, that you should never provide medical services on the basis of age, sex, race, or what have you. I want to make an exception to age—I think we really should use age as a standard, because I think it's a meaningful standard. You can't use need—it will simply not work because need is open-ended. However old you are, if your heart dies, you are in need of a transplant, and you're going to need another one when that fails—again, an infinite possibility. Everybody says treat by need because it's nondiscriminatory. However, if you have infinite resources, and you have a science that knows how to provide artificial organs, then proceed, but we don't have it, and we're not likely to have it, and we're likely to bankrupt ourselves if we do have it; in any case, it's not clear that it would create a happier old age by doing those things. That's my argument for limiting health care to the elderly.

CHAPTER 5
Discussion Group Summary: The Ethics of Care and Cure with Chronically Ill Children

Jennifer Disabato

It's interesting that we ended up talking about family, because that's something that initially came to me when I thought about this discussion group. When I was reading about ethics and thinking about my own situations, it seemed to me that a good number of the moral, ethical, and legal issues related to dilemmas in health care are somewhat different with children because of the fact that children aren't able to—are not considered able to—make decisions for themselves. One of the areas I'm most interested in is the family. However, I think that as health care professionals, we find a real controversy in terms of who we necessarily advocate for, in spite of the fact that it's idealistic to think we advocate for the family as a whole.

Ten years ago we could look at the family in a slightly more defined manner, but today the family situation is such that there are many different scenarios. There are so many single-parent families; there is the step-parent family, which results in a variety of family situations; and there are homosexual partners adopting children. Obviously, there is so much variety in what kind of family we might mean when we say that word that the ethical dilemmas surrounding chronic illness and saving babies become even more complicated.

In some of my personal dilemmas in dealing with families with chronically ill children, I almost feel like one of the aspects I have become more aware of of late: there seem to be so many phases that a family goes through in these cases. You feel that a family at one point may express legitimate decisions, legitimate rights and moral reasoning upon which they're making decisions for their chronically ill child, and then two or three years down the road the principles behind those decisions and everything else have changed so much, but there is a necessity to hang on to that initial decision or let go of it for some reason. I almost feel like there are many confusing issues around families as they go through their chronicity. It appears like a developmental process: how the family feels as the years go on.

One issue I'm interested in exploring is that kind of long-term effect. The family starts out feeling one way, but they feel differently as days and months and years go on with the chronically ill child. That initial desire to do everything because "this is our child" may then change and influence how the child views him or herself as he or she becomes cognitively able to do that.

Another issue I'm curious about is how chronicity affects the objectivity of the caregivers and how advocacy is impacted by looking at the rights of the parents versus those of the child. I believe we alluded to those rights that compose psychiatric-type areas with children and adolescents—the issue of when does the child have rights—but those are sometimes more legal than medical questions, and lie outside my particular expertise. Finally, I also find it interesting to talk about the whole issue of the covenant of care and the breaking of invulnerability. I think this is something worth exploring in relation to pediatrics and the children themselves. How do we feel when someone shares their experiences with us? That in itself is an interesting question. When we start talking about vulnerability, I have an idea where that came from, but it entails such a wide variety of aspects that we could talk for years and never really come to any definite answers or even verbalize feelings.

However, while individuality is a subject we all talk about in this area, the dilemma I confront with individuality is in worrying if the family or the parents have a sense of how the child can cope. Sometimes—particularly after getting to know a child—I sense an even greater dilemma in the inner world of the family versus the inner world of the child. Perhaps, as the child gets older and is more cognitively able to make decisions, something happens in his nonverbal memory.

One situation I was involved in—this was just several years ago—was the immense anger that was expressed by a child who was about 11. He was chronically ill, had been saved as a premie at birth, had many problems, and his anger was coming out toward his parents no matter how much you can say he wasn't able to understand the big picture. He knew that he was abnormal, even though his family nurtured or loved him, and even though he was mainstreamed: they did try to give him a normal life in which he could do as other kids do. But there was a lot of anger on his part toward his parents for knowing that he was really tiny when he was born—he was just feeling a lot of anger. Although he couldn't quite put the words to it, he was very mature. It is interesting when we talk about intervention, because as these children start getting older, the anger that was internalized becomes depression, while the anger that was expressed becomes violence.

Again, I think my whole sense of this is, how do we look at it individually, and how do we separate out that inner world of the child from the inner world of the family? That is one of the things that strikes me when I hear people say that we are born alone, live alone, and die alone. We always put the concept of the family in there, but I always wonder about that individual spirit and soul of the child and where they're at in relationship to what decisions the parents have made.

Finally, it is very important that families with these problems know there is someone for them to turn to who understands the situation and to know that there are other people as well who will understand some of the decisions that they have to make. Such a situation automatically impacts the family in a manner that is on the surface very similar to the effect that occurs when any family member becomes a focal point because of illness. It doesn't matter whether that illness is alcoholism, prescription drug abuse, or anything else—the same kinds of dynamics can occur in that family.

But those cases in which you have an opportunity of improving the situation—such as those involving an alcoholic who has the possibility of working on the road to recovery—*are* different. In the case of a chronically ill child, you have a situation in which the child is not only chronically ill, but one in which the family is suffering from a chronic dysfunction because there is no possibility of that youngster getting well. Therefore, you have all sorts of different dynamics in those families than you have in various functional kinds of families. A critical part of all this is a failure to diagnose and treat those differences.

CHAPTER 6
Discussion Group Summary: How Do You Feel at Age 84?— Caring About the Experience of Aging

Sally Gadow

There is a distinct attitude about treatment of illness and treatment of the elderly among people in the United States, and part of it, I'm sure, stems from the fact that we have never experienced a war within our borders. In England, on the other hand, they obviously have experienced such a situation, and they also have exhibited an early public concern for handicapped people—such as signs and posters in libraries and other public places—that one didn't see here until much later.

I often wondered whether some of that concern did not develop because the English people had been so directly impacted by the idea of rehabilitation after the war—just as I've wondered if their whole idea of family and their direction in the care of the elderly was not also heavily influenced by having World War II fought on their doorstep. We in the United States have not experienced anything like they have in England and so it is understandable that their views would have moved in a direction that is quite different from our own.

Nonetheless, I don't think that you can suppose that England's decision to impose an age limit on transplants, dialysis, or anything else has reflected negatively on that society's view of caring—or on its ability to care—for its older citizens. I hear nothing out of England that would suggest that they aren't just as caring, and I also hear some things that suggest they perhaps are even more caring. Perhaps because of the resources that they have conserved by not giving transplants, they are able to provide a more caring environment for people to live in; at least that's suggested in some of the literature I read. Therefore, setting those sorts of standards or criteria need not be dissonant with the idea of being very caring. But it does make me think that we're back to this sorting out of treatment from caring, and curing from caring, and all sorts of other things from caring.

The issue, of course, is that these resources are limited, and whenever you make a decision in favor of one side or group, you are also making a decision against another side or group. There is some validity to the fact that if you make a decision for age to be a criterion, that means that somebody is not going to get something in the way of treatment that he or she might need. In other words, if you have limited resources, a proactive stand for one person is a reactive stand against another. We in this country did not think in the past that we did have limited resources, and there still is much debate about exactly how limited they may actually be. But we do know that everybody can't have everything any more. And we have to begin to recognize the problems that this entails.

We often talk about different policies and the bedside perspective of families, but in this discussion it is also important to talk about the way that ideas about aging have changed. Everyone does not share the assumptions that we probably share, and that is that the elderly are indeed one and the same species with the rest of us. After all, we often get the impression that many people consider them to be some kind of an endangered species or like a group of exotic animals that is wonderfully interesting to study.

It helps frequently if a person—particularly one who is working with the chronically ill elderly—is able to relate to them as they were, perhaps, 20 years ago: what type of profession they were in, how they fulfilled their needs, what their history has been. If the caregiver can feel that way, that also helps the family to feel more at ease and to remember the good times. But this still begs the question as to who this person is now and whether he or she is fullly the person as they used to be.

We do, however, deal with these questions all the time, and sometimes it seems as if we are really giving as much care to the families as we are to the patients. This raises the further question of exactly what role the nurse should play within this ethical framework. We have talked about the doctor's position in all of this, but the doctors don't talk with the families. We are outraged when a physician passes off his responsibilities in this area, and we believe strongly that nurses could handle these matters better.

But is nursing education purporting that nurses become involved in these ethical dilemmas? Where does the nurse fit in? Are we still the support givers to the physician, family, and everybody else in the world, or will we have an active part in helping people deal with these problems?

When we do talk about ethical guidelines and principles, however, it is probably best that we look at them as if they were a new language. If you are learning French, for example, you need to learn about French, the grammar, how it's all put together, and how you say what you are going to say. And if we are going to move to a higher level of sophistication on ethics and the treatment of the elderly, we similarly have to move beyond "this is what I think" and "this is what I feel." We have to move to a different level if we are really going to communicate about it. Clearly, if you are committed to it, then you have to think about ethics as being equally important to anatomy, physiology, and pharmacology. Let us build in an ethical piece to the clinical question, because this is valid. To my mind it's similar to aspects of caring: We've got to enable other people and ourselves to learn how we integrate this into how we think, practice, teach, and do research or whatever we do, because if it's just one more thing added on to what we have to do when we get everything else done that we're supposed to do, it'll never get done.

Therefore, we have to integrate the issue of ethics into what we already do. It's something that you think about when you get started, and then, hopefully, it is something that pervades all you do while you're with your patients. But it's a long process, and it takes a long time to be comfortable saying what you believe. All these things take time, but we have to do them. They are certainly worth pursuing.

At times, I feel like there is a polarization of ideas and thoughts. Early on I said that there are some people who thought we ought to call this conference "Care versus Cure." But I argued strongly not to say that, and part of the reason is the connection between science and art and the definition of modern medicine. Look at the people who are at the forefront of physics—like David Bohm and others—who are describing their work in quite unscientific terms: for example, that subatomic particles are beginning to look like dance patterns, and so on, the same as any artist or someone who gives an inspiring, fantastic performance. It's not without intelligence that it all comes out that way; it's not an accident that somebody throws sound together, and it turns out to be a symphony. In general, there's beginning to be a synchronicity with art and science exhibited by people on the cutting edge, and we need to keep that in mind and be careful we don't depolarize ourselves.

I don't believe that there is a contradiction between science and service, or art. Basically, I think artists and scientists share many common values. One is aesthetic: We all value the beauty of the human form. There's aesthetics in that, but there also can be aesthetics in a body that's not perfect, either. We do, after all, have values that are similar to those that artists strive for—the idea that we are more than our individual tasks

and actions, just as a piece of music or a painting is more than a bunch
of notes or a splash of colors.

CHAPTER 7

Discussion Group Summary: Ethical Dilemmas in the Clinical Setting— Time Constraints, Conflicts in Interprofessional Decision Making

Marilyn A. Ray

This session is of particular interest to me, both from the point of view of being closely involved with practitioners of nursing and from my own research in critical and chronic care.

Last year I conducted research in critical care; the kind of research I do is actually on the study of human experience. Currently, I'm in the chronic care area and looking at human caring. My particular interest for the last 10 years had been in the study of human caring within complex organizations, particularly hospitals. This kind of human science research—which has a number of other names like phenomenology or the study of human experience, and hermeneutics or the interpretation of meaning—has grown from the idea of caring itself and is trying to make it more humanistic. It is a qualitative approach to research; it doesn't generate numbers. We usually try to understand with respect to the way in which people express meaning through language.

When I was engaged with the nurses in understanding the meaning of critical care, for example, the main thrust or central theme of that research came out in relationship to ethical conflicts. But it was an ethical conflict not from the point at which a nurse might be fully immobilized, but from the point at which the nurse—and those who are learning from nurses—can indeed begin to question, think, try to understand, and perhaps even change the way in which we teach problem solving.

In critical care, the major ethical conflict, of course, revolves around the uses or abuses of technology itself. When we begin to look at a critical care unit, its value is generally related to saving lives through the use of technology. That is the means by which we have the chance to save lives. What happens in these situations and what has occurred as a result of this study is that nurses talked about caring in many different ways: from a perspective of transpersonal humanistic vulnerability to a conflictual, almost dichotomist understanding of how actually to care. In these kinds of situations, those of you who work in them probably see this occurrence minute by minute. The conflict, therefore, arises out of first understanding the use of technology, what happens when a nurse or often a physician—but usually not both at the same time—begins to recognize that the technology itself is of little or no value, and what happens in terms of the decisions that occur after that.

To give you an example, we'll take the case of Mary working with Peter, who is a 75-year-old congestive heart failure patient who has had two coronaries in the past and has been admitted to the intensive care unit. He is not responding to treatment, and it looks as though his worsening condition will not be reversible by the use of technology. In this case, Mary, by virtue of what she really believes about technology, thinks that the respirator and the other kinds of pharmacological treatments that we use in critical care are no longer helping. But she—being a human being who is interacting with someone else as a human being—is not just treating that person as an object. She is a feeling person who is taking on an empathic suffering relationship with this patient in terms of understanding what to do in a situation like this.

What this means is that there is a point in working in critical care where a sort of movement exists from ethical conflict through ethical dilemma to ethical crisis. And that is occurring in practice all the time. Sometimes a nurse may be in conflict with a particular treatment that the physician has ordered, or it might actually be a dilemma that's in conflict with one's own belief system in terms of the kind of treatment that is going on, but it has thrown the health care professional—or primarily in this case, the nurse—into a crisis of decision. As a result, through ethical conflict decisions are sometimes made for the patient that bring about a great deal of suffering for the patient and family as well as for the nurse and also the physician.

In these studies, I've found that while the nurse, indeed, has developed a bonding relationship with the patient, someone who is being worked with very closely, and within that context of vulnerability and bonding, the kinds of suffering that exist are not always terminated. Sometimes nurses keep it within themselves and don't always share, but they find that new decisions have to be made for the patient. On the other hand, often the physician does not form a sensitive, close bonding, and caring relationship with the patient, so the kinds of decisions that need to be made are not made soon enough.

Sometimes the decision to do something takes too long to formulate, even though the nurse knows it should have been done almost immediately. That puts the nurse in a crisis state for quite a while. There is a recognizable pattern to this: The nurse will begin dealing with the conflict herself or himself, and then you begin to see the interaction with others. Sometimes that's right away; and then it moves to another level of hierarchy. Then sometimes nurses can't address the attending physician directly, and so this process, I've found, sometimes takes more than three days and could take seven to ten days. The physician, most of the time, is not the one who can be dealt with directly in this situation, so the nurse has to go through much maneuvering in order to get new decisions made when she herself has identified that the technologies, whether they are pharmacology or some kind of intervention by machine, no longer are doing any good. And she has to deal with the conflict related to family or spouse, so that whole system can throw a unit into a crisis situation.

What I am proposing is that we change the way we've taught the nursing process—which has been primarily through an objective problem-solving realm—so that we deal with it through an ethical decision-making process. We must use a type of ethical inquiry in relationship to the notion of the concept of bonding itself between the nurse and the patient, and the problem of distance between the doctor and the patient in those kinds of situations, and then from that understanding determine what happens in terms of outcome: what kinds of decisions are made as a result of that. I call part of that a type of transactional ethic, which is beginning to look at the response of the nurse and the patient, and then the ways the nurse moves from an understanding of what is happening to the points at which she can follow principles of ethics.

That is the kind of system that I see evolving from the intensive care unit, at least in the study that I was working on. But since I've presented it in many places, I continue to get confirmation that we must have understanding of nursing through a problem-solving or objective point in which we identify the problem, manage the problem, and evaluate the problem. Quite simply, this puts us outside the realm of the processes that are actually going on, which are bonding and responding through that bonding to the point that we can begin within ourselves to try to make sense out of what is moral within us and what is the right thing to do. Those are the kinds of things that I see creating both the intrapersonal conflict and the interprofessional conflict.

CHAPTER 8
Discussion Group Summary: Grounded in Self, in Both Caring and Curing

Francelyn Reeder

I'd like to give you a framework. By this I mean one of your free choices is to look at the self as the ground from which you, an individual person—whether you're a patient or a nurse, or just any individual in life—can base all decisions, no matter what they are, no matter whether they are ethical or a matter of taste. The ultimate court of appeals always rests with you, so I'd like to draw you to a certain disposition and way of looking at yourself as the source of the ultimate decision.

We have ethics and norms, and, consequently, policies, protocols, and lots of people telling us what are the best ways to do things and for what reasons. All of that information somehow or other from childhood on up has to be processed and assimilated, and we also believe in having to make the decision ourselves. It can often be a lonely decision, even in the midst of people; the decision you have to make is yours. Therefore, what I'd like to do is just give you a framework for doing that and talk about some specific examples where we could see how this operates.

This brings a dilemma to mind in terms of what I'm going to share with you; we will talk about it and see what your point of view is. But first let me just ask if anyone has had any experience of centering or deep meditative prayer, no matter what tradition you follow. Have you ever heard the phrases "get grounded," "get it together," or "find the core of your being"? Different people come to different readings, traditions, etc. These all mean the same thing in my mind, and I come from a background of philosophy, phenomenology, and identifying where you go when you center, or what is this sense of being at home. It's

41

another way of asking what is the ground of my being, the core, the deep seat and what is most to me if you take anything away from me? If I lose a limb, if I lose an eye, what about me is really me? Some people call that being in tune, as well. There's a foundation to which we can go that we can call home, and just for a minute I'd like to invite you to sit comfortably. I want to take just five minutes to help you get into this position of reaching whatever you call home, and then we will discuss that and put it in the frame. Because if you can't find that place, then what I'm going to talk about will not mean much, but it will certainly be a conversation piece. However, I want to give you the chance of reaching down deep in yourself. So just find it quiet, get comfortable, close your eyes if you want, and I'll take you verbally down to the center of your own being.

Take in a couple of deep breaths, close your eyes, get comfortable, drop the concerns of the day, feel yourself in your chair. Take in a deep breath and blow it out and listen to your body; listen to your consciousness; smell the breeze, and flow with it. Let go, and flow with what you feel. Get a sense of becoming, coming in deeper to yourself, and flowing off. Pay attention to any images that come into your mind, any sensations, any auditory sounds, whether it's music or just the throbbing of your own heart, or the rhythm of your respirations. Now take another deep breath and sink down deep within until you reach a point of being calm. Continue to breathe deep and let it out. Whatever place you have found yourself in your images or musical sounds, follow it, don't fight it . . . trust it, flow with it, embrace it, drink it in. Call it your own. This is your space, your place, being at home. While you swell in it, without losing contact and embracing that space, let your awareness just be expansive. Don't worry about which way it's going. Take in another deep breath, drink it in, call it your own. Wherever you feel comfortable—that peaceful place, go with it, listen to it, listen to anything that comes to you. Respect it, trust it, let it go if it is fleeing away. Something else is coming in place of it. Look at it, embrace it, continue breathing. While feeling that sensation, move around just a little bit, slowly, while retaining that feeling of being at home, wiggle around a little, open your eyes if you like. Recall that you are in this room, in this chair, with this group of people, enjoy . . . . Now try to sustain that sense of feeling at home. There isn't any right or wrong way of feeling, so everyone's experiences are legitimate.

All of us have some things in common and some things that are very uniquely ours, and we also have indicated that there's been a pattern. Some of us return to the same places. We can, at will, choose to feel a certain way by doing that. Once we experience our inner selves and choose to find a peaceful place within our own cores, we become more used to knowing how we can do that, and just the simple taking of time for practice away from others is critical. Later on, when we get into that mode, even in the workaday world, we can intentionally decide to do that. When we're walking down the hall, for instance, we can give ourselves 30 seconds of being in that place, of being centered on the way, and it does take away from our busy world. And I want to put it in another framework that gives us some confidence and substantial reaffirmation from many philosophers' points of view as to the basic structure of consciousness of the world, our inner connectiveness with the world. No matter who it is that we speak to and no matter how much education people have, if they do get into themselves, if they find their center, if they return to the ground of their being, which is that most personal place often called home, these are some of the kinds of things they will describe. And the framework I'm going to describe, I would say, is the same place we need to go when we are making decisions, no matter what type they are. It's a way of knowing whether we are just a reed in the wind, getting on every bandwagon that comes along, or new trend or whatever—that when that comes along, this place we call home is what we need to pull up and get a sense of. Then we judge this new thing that comes along against our own center, because in choosing what's coming along it should be integral with ourselves, and if it isn't, it somehow or other doesn't feel like being at home. This takes practice. Then it is something that we stay in doubt of, and we just don't get on the bandwagon. Ethical decision making involves doing this very thing, even more critically. But let me offer a slight framework and see what this says.

After having centered, and I invite you to the depths of your being, to the ground of your being, phenomenology would say where you go is to the very structure of your consciousness that many of you talk about anticipating, some of you talk about remembering. In any given moment in the present, we have a past that we can recall, where we've just left. As I speak this word, it becomes a memory to you, because I'm saying another word, and another and another word. So my words flow off and become memory, but you don't forget them as I speak. You then know and get a sense—you can anticipate that I'm going to complete the sentence, and this is a sense of a future coming, something coming. All of you have that dynamic flow. You can put in these words. Perhaps an ordinary way of saying it in phenomenology is that these are retentions. These experiences you had are retained. They don't go away. I'm speaking primarily to your awareness and your consciousness of expansion, and in the present, there's always a flow in. If you can focus and be in touch with your very core, often in the core you have past, present, and the future. It's not split off.

What we often call illness is when people can't remember the past and don't have a sense of the future. They feel isolated and disconnected. Think about teenagers and the suicide rate going up; the very thing that happens is that they don't remember their past. It isn't so important to remember the details of the past, but that they have a past. There's a continuity within you, and it's worthwhile returning to it, knowing it, and becoming familiar with it. Similarly, we have a future. There's no dead end. Part of the way you look at the present is to know that the future is opening up, not necessarily being always created by you, but one that is being created in your very living perhaps at a more primordial, unconscious level, and aspects of it that are created by you and chosen by you. But even before you get to the level of a choice, a primordial awareness of having a past, present, and future is there. It's part of our being.

CHAPTER 9
Discussion Group Summary:
Family and Community Dimensions of the
Ethics of Care with Chronically Ill Persons

Phyllis Schultz

and Robert Schultz

All people in the nursing profession tend to get tied up to some extent in their own feelings in regard to the treatment regimen of their patients. Also, an individual's education may help to determine—at least to a degree—how they respond to patient care. Many actually become detached or removed from the situation because they feel that doing so allows them to render better care and prevents too much involvement with the patient. But others contend that this does not work, because nurses do a better job if they are directly involved in the sense that they become acutely aware of the various choices that are open to those for whom they are caring.

Respecting patients' right to choose is a difficult stance for most health care providers, however, for most of them have known of patients who said they would not follow the recommendations of their physicians—and also of physicians who could not deal with that reaction. They would give all kinds of excuses as to why this was inappropriate for the patient, but what was really meant was that it was inappropriate for the patient to refuse to follow physician recommendations. But other health care professionals are beginning to concede that this would indeed be appropriate if the patient's decision was based upon his or her desire to spare

This paper was prepared with the collaboration of Howard Rothman, member of the American Medical Writers Association, Rockville, MD.

the family from the financial strain that would result from such a treatment procedure. Some support this type of decision while others do not, and it causes a great deal of conflict among providers.

One of the effects of a stance like the above is to make caregivers feel vulnerable. It tells them that what they have to give is not good enough; it makes the caring situation awkward.

Another circumstance that can compound the problem is when patients believe that the quality of life ahead would not be worth the living. It may not be what they wanted, and so even if they do not verbalize it, the knowledge that their situation was very restricted and would become only more so over time might play a major part in a decision.

There is, in this case, also the choice between care that will prolong life at various kinds of costs: costs to the family's resources, costs to the family's ability to get on with their lives, costs to the patient in terms of suffering. And the question always remains whether the prolonging of life, even with the possibility of continuing relationships, comes out positive in the balancing of benefits and costs.

Two very important problems in this equation, however, remain largely unanswered. One is the manner in which such conflicts are dealt with once they arise; the other is that such conflicts do not exist in isolation, but are part and parcel of what is going on in the community and in society as a whole. Emotions play a large part in both of these problems, but emotions are often looked down upon as a female trait while the decision making and action part of the situation is often looked upon as the male role. Even though nurses are talking about caring, ethics, and dilemmas in their practice, it is very often the male physicians who are directing the choices and performing the technological acrobatics while their largely female nursing counterparts are left to deal with the emotional support of the patient and family. As long as these two areas—decision making and emotional support—are separated, society will continue experiencing emotional upheavals as families are split apart by the oftentimes conflicting desires of patients, physicians, nurses, and the community at large.

How comfortable, for example, would most nurses be in initiating a conversation with a doctor by saying that since a patient is going to die—or at least that the likelihood of that happening is very strong—how can we and the family best handle the situation? Frequently, even if such a conversation is begun, the physician will not have much of an answer. The nurse will ask why, since so-and-so is doing badly, are we doing this for him? The physician may answer that it is all for the family, so again it returns to the issues already noted.

On the other hand, what about a joint conference that would be attended by the physician, the nurse, the family, and maybe even the patient? That would probably be the last resort; most providers would much prefer to have it taken care of in some sort of one-on-one discussion or else through an intermediary. In addition, it's very difficult to arrange a meeting like that on an emergency basis. But there are models and procedures for such a conference—including those in which the physician is not present, and others which may be attended by the nursing staff, the dietician, and even the chaplain.

Some wonder why it should be so much trouble to call together a conference that deals with the very issues that are paramount to why such health care professionals care for people in the first place. It is difficult, others note, because it takes physicians and other caretakers away from their immediate jobs, but also because of the politics involved, which may be insurmountable.

All of these issues, however, revolve continually around the question of vulnerability, which may be the most important factor in the equation. Caregivers tend to get angry when patients want to take control, because that increases their vulnerability—and that is something most cannot deal with in their own intimate relationships, much less in regard to someone whom they don't really even know. Families also have a hard time letting go because it renders the whole family unit, as well as most of its individual components, vulnerable, and people just cannot allow themselves easily to become weak. They believe instead that they must remain strong and invulnerable.

Additionally, it is apparent that the family and the health care providers would probably make different decisions at different points in time, so if one is not dealing with a chronically or terminally ill person who is eventually going to die, there is no real need for an immediate decision. A one-shot conference would then not provide the ultimate answer, in part because the people involved are going to be coming along at different rates of speed and are going to be accepting the reality of the situation at different levels and at different points. Perhaps, by expecting to come up with a miracle decision in a split second, we're actually pulling together a group in which nobody is prepared to make the ultimate decision. Perhaps the emotions would come along with the science and the curing if the situation was examined longitudinally and was left to unfold over time.

Finally, those in the nursing profession often express a profound feeling of powerlessness in situations involving ethical dilemmas. But many still profess a desire to initiate some kind of method or procedure for resolving such a conflict, even if they feel stymied by a strongly bureaucratic orientation—either in terms of the organization's administration or in terms of medical control. It's one thing to be in an institution where there is an ethics committee that can be approached and another to be in a setting where no such structure exists and where nurses feel particularly powerless. What is happening across the country may be improvement, but it remains largely a situation where nurses feel unable to act on what they believe is right in terms of their own practice. Some may handle the matter by announcing that they will not provide care in a situation they do not feel is appropriate, but most of them realize that this is not the easiest thing to do.

CHAPTER 10
Discussion Group Summary: Personal versus Professional Ethical Dilemmas

Anna Seroka

I want to provide you with a very brief background in ethical decision making; but I hope, by this, to be able to exhibit something of the framework behind personal types of ethical conflicts. Unless you begin to understand the causes of ethical conflicts, you will have a hard time understanding why certain ethical decisions are made.

One of the things that I do want to outline is the process for decision making. It's a very simple process: It's identifying alternatives, evaluating those alternatives, choosing the appropriate alternative, and then carrying out your decision. And that seems very, very simple. So why, when it comes to ethics, do we have so many problems? How many of you get very frustrated when ethical decisions are made? Now I'm not going to give you anything black and white to help you understand that, but hopefully I am going to have you look into yourselves so that you know why some of these decisions are made.

One of the first things we see, or one of the first reasons that there is no black and white as far as ethical decision making, is that we have two major theories of ethics and two major principles: One is utilitarian, and one is deontological. Now these are two very acceptable theories upon which you make your ethical decisions. If you are a utilitarian and you are making an ethical decision, what you are looking at is what is good for the utility or for the majority, not the individual. When you're looking from the stance of a deontologic person, and you're making an ethical decision, you're looking at it from what is best for the individual, what are the rights of the individual—not necessarily what is good for the majority.

Let me provide you with a practical example: There's a family that consists of a father who is its sole support, a mother, a 2-year-old son, a 10-year-old daughter, and a 14-year-old son. The 14-year-old is diagnosed as having end-stage renal disease, and in need of a transplant. You know that, when you're transplanting organs, the best donor is a member of the family as far as doing your tissue typing, etc. In this situation, the father was the best donor for his son. However, when you take a kidney from someone, that leaves him or her with one kidney, and statistics have shown that this, in many cases, substantially reduces the life span; plus, there is the potential that if something happens to that one kidney, then you've created an end-stage renal disease patient, and you have the same problem as before.

The physician involved looked at this case from a deontologic stance and said to the father, "You are the absolute best donor for your son. Your son has a right to the best choice of organs." That doesn't mean he couldn't have gotten an organ from an organ bank; he certainly could have. However, because the organ was not from a relative, the son might have rejected it sooner. The physician's stance was that the son has a right to this kidney. The father now looked at it from the utilitarian standpoint and said, "I have a 2-year-old and a 10-year-old, and my wife doesn't work. Now my wife is not skilled in any particular work area, and if anything happens to me, she would have to support them. But in order to make enough money she would have to work harder than I would want her to, because she doesn't have any special job skills." So he looked at it from the utilitarian standpoint, and of course in the situation there was a tremendous argument, with the physician saying deontologically, your son has a right to the best, and the father saying, but I have to look at what's best for the majority. Who's right?

What I'm trying to show you now is why, just based on ethical theory, there is not always a right or a wrong. Have I made that point? There is another critical factor in decision making, which may begin to enter into what you're saying or why you're saying he's wrong. Let me just ask you to identify what the other critical factor is, because I'm not going to tell you now. I'm going to see if you can tell me.

When we're talking about decision making, we're talking about a very simple process. And it's not even ethical decision making; you do this with every decision that you make. But with ethics we add in these theories, so they enter into our ethical decision making, and then we begin to look at things from different frameworks: the patient, the institution that we work in, and self. When we start looking at self, we really do start looking at values.

Now you can talk to many people who say that by the time you're 10 years old, you've established your values. I have to say that's practically true but not until after babies do what they call imprinting. People just make an impression on them, they imprint. Role-modeling is the next stage you go through, and that happens during adolescence up to about 12 or 13 years old. Before you hit your teens, you have that motivation for role-modeling. You know, what do you want to be when you grow up; who do you want to be like? There's always a hero or a role model, and many people feel it is during that time when you do establish your values. And I think you do establish a value system during that time, because you sure don't establish it when you're in your teens. In your teens you're too busy fighting all those values; that's your period of socialization. Now you need to go out and if it's what you want to do socially, if to be like everybody else interferes with values you've learned during your role-modeling period, you're in trouble. You express significant conflict, and you begin to fight backward and forward. Hopefully, by the time you're in your 20s, you have made some decision as to what values you're going to keep and what values you're going to give up.

However, I disagree with sociologists when they say you've formed your values at 10 years of age. I disagree because I can think, just even in my own personal experiences, as you begin to change things in your life, as you begin to live with different cultures, as you begin to move into different professions, as you begin to move to different parts of the country, you begin to look at things very differently. There are some values that you keep, there are some values that you give up just because you've broadened your experiences in life. Yet what I need to say is that you do have values. Anyone who says he or she doesn't have values is lying; he or she *does* have them, whatever they are. The older you get, the less they change, but there is still some room for change as you go through life. If your life changes a lot, your values will change. Contrarily, if you come from the North End in Boston, which is the Italian section, and never move out of that area, I guarantee you, your values probably won't change. But you can go from there to California and meet a whole different type of population and people, and you'll begin to take what meets your needs best from that new population, and bring that into your own value system.

A significant part of the issue of personal ethical conflict versus professional ethical conflict is that you can't really separate the two, not at all. What you have to be able to do is to look at where you're coming from and stand back. It's almost like asking, "Where am I coming from?": basically what you're doing is a values clarification. Just quickly ask in your mind, "Where am I coming from? Is this for me or is it for the patient?" Once you realize where you're coming from, you almost need to pick that up and say to yourself, "And now, I know where I'm coming from; now I need to look at where the patient is coming from." If you can't do that, then you need help from the family and from perhaps other people . . . . the chaplain, people on the ethics committee, etc.

CHAPTER 11
Discussion Group Summary:
When Caring Doesn't Mean Curing

Father Paul Wicker

One of the central questions that comes up often in nursing work is whether or not healing can occur without cure. This, of course, involves delving into parts of a patient's being that have little to do with his or her actual physical state. Also it comes on top of two other kinds of related situations: the one in which people experience some type of condition that may get in their way once in a while even though they are by no means truly ill, and the one in which people suffer from a chronic illness that simply cannot be cured. Both of these situations, nonetheless, still fall within the context of caring, even if there is actually no curing involved. And both of these situations illustrate that absolute positions are not always the only issues of importance.

Caring, many agree, is a way of helping the patient to bring his or her whole life into balance, and it can occur whether or not true curing takes place. A perfect example can be found within the psychiatric field. There, many professionals set their sights solely on caring even when they do not believe that a cure can take place.

Another part of this overall issue involves the health care professional's ability to facilitate certain patients to become aware of what their own resources might be, so that they can see how much care they can give to themselves and their own families. This ability can help the patient to discover what his or her own capacities are—and the initial act of caring can also evolve into an act of curing for the patient as well as his family.

But does the very concept of "caring" always assume that an illness must be present in the first place? Curing certainly does, as it is intended to move someone from illness to wellness. But caring need not: It can instead involve caring for a loved one, or, in the nurse–patient relationship, caring for the wellness of that individual instead of just his or her illness.

Caring, then, should perhaps be separated from its usual relationship with a specific disease, because that often leads to the division of a patient into disease and object and the ultimate caring for only that person's disease. If the health care professional shifts gears so as to be caring for a person with a disease instead, then perhaps this can allow for the concentration of caring for wellness and the source of life. This also may have the benefit of permitting the professional to be less tempted to become disembodied.

It also can be helpful in treating those people who are not necessarily ill, but who have some type of psychological distress that could eventually lead to illness. All of us have probably utilized this way of thinking in our personal lives, such as when family members or friends came under tremendous stress or received some shocking news. We've proven on a regular basis that people can get through incredible periods of emotional upheaval if they are given adequate support and caring, and we automatically offer this type of diseaseless caring process to young children and older persons. It just may not be offered in big enough doses to other adults on a regular basis.

It may not be entirely possible, however, to completely escape the disease model or the illness model when discussing this subject. Caring could, in other words, still be seen as a process of moving one person from a state of incompleteness to a state of completeness, which is another way of saying from a state of dis-ease to a state of ease. It can be illustrated by considering the common experience of those health care professionals who refuse to step forcefully into their own medical care processes even if they are knowledgeable about things that should be done. This stems in part from the fact that the very act of becoming a patient renders most of us back to basics, almost back to a childlike state of being. For those who surrender to this basic human condition, a little bit of encouragement—a little bit of caring—can help tremendously in putting their self-determination back on track.

Caring without curing also becomes a viable and common occurrence following a death, particularly one that strikes a family unaccustomed to dealing with such tragedies. For someone experiencing their first funeral, for example, the mechanics of where to go, what to pay, and how to get it all done quickly while still in a state of confusion and grief can be seriously overwhelming. A friend, perhaps a nurse who was treating the deceased, can help the bereaved to move through this difficult period more easily by a simple heartfelt act of caring.

Consider the case of a 3-year-old boy who died of a brain tumor that was diagnosed at 1 year of age. It had been a very trying situation for the parents, and even the nurses involved were helpless to some degree. Most—as might be expected—felt vulnerable and exposed in their dealings with the family, and especially in trying to explain to them that the caregivers really could not be of any medical help because death was inevitable. The parents were, after all, aware of the situation's grimness on one level, but it was on that other, completely emotional level, that medical personnel always trained toward the goal of physical cure were bewildered. Nonetheless, after curing was no longer possible and the little boy died, the act of caring for the grieving parents still continued. There were a number of people from the hospital and the hospice who took time out from their own lives to be present at the funeral—and that showed to the parents in no uncertain terms exactly how much they did care. It also illustrates full well how health care professionals can care and reach out to people long past the point where any sort of physical or external cure is possible. Their mere presence said more than many a word.

Undoubtedly, it is easy to get into the mode that if there is no cure possible, then maybe all that can still take place is custodial care. Those in the nursing profession, however, can still assist these patients—as well as their families—by helping them to first experience what life does remain as fully as possible, and then by offering aid and comfort to the surviving family members. However, this is complicated somewhat by a system that does not always allow for all of such options to be utilized. In the case of those who suffer from Parkinson's or Alzheimer's disease, for example, physical therapy that might make the patient feel more comfortable is not always valid because it does not cure and thus may not be covered by insurance. Yet these patients really need this type of attention, almost more than anything else in terms of keeping them moving and functional and comfortable. This adds one more ethical question to the overall debate.

A balance, it seems, is the ultimate solution. Caring doesn't always mean curing, although it is true that both often go hand-in-hand. Support networks, patient advocates, and other integrated systems all can help those who need them to get through rough times when no actual illness may be present. All of us need such caring at some points in our lives, and it is the fortunate few who are lucky enough to receive it.